Healing Wines & Syrups

Excerpted from
The Herbal Home Remedy Book,
by Joyce A. Wardwell

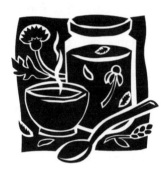

CONTENTS

Introduction

My great-grandmother Na never went to a doctor in her life. She dismissed doctors as charlatans, saw their medicines as harmful, and thought hospitals were places you went to die. Her back-then attitudes weren't that much different from our attitudes today, only now we mistrust shifty HMOs, spiraling hospital bills, and the side effects of drugs. Just like my grandmother, we believe that "I can do it better." One of the most famous doctors of this century, Albert Schweitzer, expressed exactly this sentiment: "It's supposed to be a professional secret, but I'll tell you anyway. We doctors do nothing. We only help and encourage the doctor within."

Indeed, roughly 80 percent of the world's population uses traditional medicine for primary health care. And lest you doubt the effectiveness of plant remedies, realize that about 30 percent of prescription drugs are still synthesized from plants. As we enter the 21st century, Na's attitude toward medicine is experiencing an amazing rebirth, even in our high-tech Western culture. An increasing array of commercially prepared herbal remedies faces me whenever I enter the drugstore. There are even whole commercial chains devoted to selling the cures that wise women and men have been making themselves for centuries!

More and more clever people continue to do so today, and that's where this book comes in. Herbal preparations can be as much of a pleasure to consume as they are to make. Why choke down factory-made pills with water like any prescription when you can take your medicine in a civilized glass of wine? Why force some artificially flavored cough elixir into your daughter when you could give her a lavender- or lemon-flavored one that will soothe her raw throats as well? And even more important, why disregard powerful herbal allies in our quest for good health?

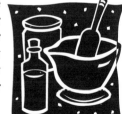

Caution

Like any medicine, it is important to use herbs with care. The simple herbal recipes in this booklet are meant to inspire, and they are not given as medical advice. For your individual health concerns, for chronic warning symptoms, in emergency situations, or when in doubt, seek the advice of your primary health-care practitioner.

As you will see, all you need in order to make your own herbal remedies is the following:

- A few pieces of equipment you may already own
- Access to fresh or dried medicinal herbs
- Liquids and sweeteners (known as base ingredients) to carry the herbs into your body
- Time and care to put into your project

You will be amply rewarded with some delightful foodstuffs and elixirs, many of which can become part of your daily routine.

Basic Equipment:
As Close as Your Kitchen

The equipment you use to make your remedies will affect how they turn out. The good news is that home herbalism requires no special distillers, tubes, condensers, or other supplies. Chances are that you have everything you need already — or can find it at a garage sale for next to nothing.

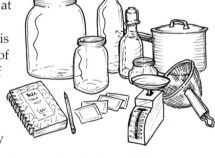

Notebook. A blank notebook is one of your most important pieces of equipment. Be sure to keep track of your favorite recipes, references, and suppliers' addresses and telephone numbers. Because I gather or grow nearly all of my herbs, I also note the seasonal and daily weather conditions, gathering dates, and places. I

You may already have all the equipment you need right in your kitchen.

write notes and observations about the preparation process. I even write down my mistakes — they are valuable little lessons that I don't wish to repeat.

Labels. However large or small, fancy or plain, labels are the herbalist's best friend. Use them relentlessly: A remedy is not finished until it has a label on it. At the very least, list the ingredients and the date. Other helpful items to note include what the preparation is for, how it should be used, how it should be stored, and where the herbs were obtained.

Cheesecloth. This white or natural-colored gauzy fabric is available in a variety of thread counts, making looser or tighter fabric. It is used in food preparation to strain and press liquids from solids — in the case of cheese, to squeeze the whey from the curds that will become cheese, and in the case of wine and vinegar, to press every last drop of tea from brewed herbs. It can also be layered into a filter to help maintain purity. It is available in kitchen supply stores in plastic packages that contain a couple of yards.

Glass jars. Colored glass jars and bottles with lids are treasures to any herbalist. Check out your local recycling station for free jars. A local restaurant-bar lets me haul away as many empty liquor and wine bottles and 1-gallon pickle jars as I care to. Saturday night offers me the best selection. Secondhand shops always have interesting finds, usually for less than a dime apiece.

Disinfecting Bottles and Jars

Disinfect all bottles, jars, and equipment before you use them by boiling them for 10 minutes or by rinsing them with a 3 percent hydrogen peroxide solution, commonly available at grocery stores and pharmacies. If you choose peroxide, begin by simply washing your equipment with soap and water, then rinsing. Pour a small amount of peroxide into the jar, shake vigorously, and drain. Finally, rinse with water and air-dry.

Scale. A small diet scale is a useful piece of equipment to have on hand for making herbal remedies, since weight is a more precise unit of measure than volume. For most mild herbs, the medicinal dose is 1 ounce (28 g) of herb to 32 ounces (950 ml) of water. Because an ounce of dried leaves has greater volume than an ounce of roots, most beginners find it helpful to use a scale until they become accustomed to the proportions.

Strainer and press. To strain a cup of tea, any stainless-steel sieve works well. But as you'll notice, when you strain you lose a lot of precious liquid from the loose herbs. This is valuable medicine. A press works much better than a strainer for these purposes.

A quick and effective homemade press can be assembled easily from a lid that fits inside a small jar. Apply wrist pressure to the lid to squeeze out as much liquid extract as possible. I have also found that food mills — the kind used to strain baby food — give satisfying results. But for the best extraction it's hard to beat a winepress.

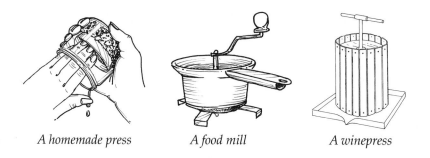

A homemade press   *A food mill*   *A winepress*

This piece of equipment is common. inexpensive, and easy to use. You can find one at kitchen accessory stores or beer- and winemaking suppliers. Do tell them that you are using it only for home herbal use lest they try to sell you a commercial grape crusher!

Mortar and pestle. If you're going to buy only one piece of special equipment for making herbal remedies, this is the one to buy. Using a mortar and pestle to grind dried roots, leaves, and seeds is the only way you can be assured that your herb powder will be fresh. If you live near a flowing creek, you can look to any little waterfalls for natural stone mortars made of quartz or basalt. I have a stone slab that serves as my mortar; using a fist-size round rock as my pestle makes for extra-quick grinding.

Herbs can also be ground efficiently in a hand-cranked coffee grinder set aside just for this purpose. (Don't use it to make coffee afterward, or your coffee will taste like the herbs!) And even though electric coffee grinders may seem more efficient, try to avoid them. The herbs get too hot, which destroys delicate oils and essences. Still, if the convenience of an electric grinder is important to you, try freezing the herbs first, then grinding small batches in short bursts only. This should keep the herbs from getting hot.

Choosing the Right Equipment

Every piece of equipment that comes in contact with the herbal preparations should be as nonreactive as possible. An herbal extract made in an aluminum pot will contain aluminum residue. On the other hand, glass, unchipped enamel, stainless steel, and marble are all excellent nonreactive materials. Likewise, unbleached muslin, Lucite cutting boards, and wooden spoons are all desirable.

Base Ingredients and Carriers

These are the basic ingredients we'll be discussing in this bulletin. Following is a description of each ingredient, along with advice on how to ensure purity and the highest quality for each.

Wines

Don't use commercial wines for medicine making. Wine grapes are heavily sprayed with fungal and mold inhibitors, and sulfites and cadmium are used to make the wine. Studies have also shown that the foil wrapper often used around a bottle's seal can leak lead into the wine. For medicinal wines, you need to make your own. Turn to page 15 for recipes and instructions.

Vinegars

A good-quality vinegar is alive. Vinegar is made by inoculating wine with "mother vinegar" — bacteria. A living vinegar is slightly cloudy, and there is a sediment on the bottom of the bottle. You can buy apple cider vinegar with the mother in it at most health food stores, but it is a bit pricey. Making your own vinegar is easy and fun — see the directions that begin on page 26.

Honey

Buy honey that is free of pesticides and contaminants. By and large I find that beekeepers with small-scale operations avoid using sprays — perhaps because beekeeping by its very nature involves an understanding of nature's web.

Try to buy honey grown close to your home. Each country — indeed, each county — produces a distinct type of honey. People with hay fever or allergies sometimes find relief from eating locally produced honey. Stop in at your local farmer's market and find a person who is selling crystallized honey, which is raw and unfiltered. Raw honey contains enzymes that have antibiotic abilities — enzymes that are destroyed by light and heat, making raw honey your best choice for medicinal use. I think it tastes better as well. There are people who swear by the superior qualities of dark honey; medicinally, I find little difference between dark and light, however.

Caution

The Centers for Disease Control in Atlanta recommends that raw honey should not be served to children under 1 year old. You may want to play it safe and avoid giving honey to children for their first two years. Some uncooked honeys may contain botulism spores that are harmless to older children and adults, but can cause a fatal diarrhea in an immature digestive system.

Sugars

Sugars are used to make wines and syrups and to sweeten bitter brews. Alternatives to refined white table sugar include honey (see above) and maple syrup. Maple syrup contains trace minerals that are carried up in a tree's sap from as much as 60 feet (18 m) below the ground. A pure maple syrup has a flowery aroma and buttery texture. Grade A Amber syrup comes from the first flow of sap and is considered the best by some, though others prefer the richer flavor and darker color of Grade B. Medicinally, it is a matter of personal preference.

Another sweetening alternative is stevia, an herbal sweetener that has been used worldwide for centuries but has been available in the United States only since 1988. The U.S. Food and Drug Administration has not approved stevia as a sweetener, only as a food additive. It's up to 300 times sweeter than sugar; use just 1 teaspoon (5 ml) of stevia in place of 1 cup (237 ml) of sugar. Its sweetening ability is similar to that of sucrose, with little aftertaste. Stevia has a fleeting flavor, reminiscent of honeysuckle, that seems to disappear in tea or cooking. Another positive factor is that stevia is not a nutrition source for oral bacteria; in fact, it actually helps suppress cavities!

Which Herbs to Use?

An herb's quality determines its healing capacity. Would you eat a salad made from wilted brown lettuce or dried lettuce greens? Certainly not by choice. If it were served in a restaurant, you'd demand a refund. Yet we pay for poor-quality herbs wrapped in expensive high-quality packages all the time. To ensure that we have the best herbal medicine, we must train ourselves to look beyond the wrapping and into the herb itself.

Given all possible choices, I always choose the fresh herb. The fresh plant has a vitality that quickly degrades. Studies done by the Rodale Institute show that a head of broccoli left out in the sun can lose as much as half of its vitamin C content in the first half hour! In the refrigerator, nutrient loss slows but still occurs. Careful herbalists gather or grow their own herbs whenever possible to ensure the best quality.

Caring for the Harvest

Whether you forage for herbs in the wild or raise your own, plan to prepare them for storage immediately after you gather them. Herbs left to sit even overnight will degrade in quality. Shake off the dirt. Sort out dead leaves and debris. Separate stems from leaves and seeds from chaff. Wash and blot dry roots, then spread them out to dry. Roots will need to be chopped into pieces about 1 inch (2.5 cm) thick; leaves and flowers are best left as whole as possible. There are many ways to preserve your harvest: Drying and freezing are just two of the options you may wish to pursue in addition to making the herbal remedies discussed here.

Buying Your Herbs

Of course it isn't always possible to have your own herb garden and grow every plant you would like to, in the quantity you want. If this is your situation, it is usually fine to use a dried, purchased product. Always get the freshest dried herbs you can. Although dried herbs last longer than fresh, they do continue to gradually lose their essential oils — and with them their scent, flavor, and ability to heal. The best place to find bulk herbs is in natural food stores.

Storage Tips

To keep a watchful eye on your stored herbs, consider keeping them in clear glass jars. Then you can easily see any color changes — a sure sign of corruption. Just be certain to keep the jars in the dark behind a curtain or door.

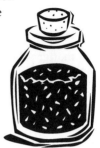

Sunlight, air, heat, moisture, and reactive metals such as aluminum, tin, and copper are the enemies of your stored herbs. They slowly corrupt the herbs' vitality and potency. It is best to store your herbs in a cool, dark, and ventilated area such as a kitchen cabinet, pantry, or cellar.

The Spirit of Medicinal Herbalism

The essence of herbal medicine is the quest for balance. Simply put, balance as a chronic state evokes health. Aristotle named it *moderation* and said, "Man must enjoy his moderation, lest that, too, become excessive." At their best, medicinal plants become part of daily living, our food, thus preventing our tendency to swing from one extreme to another.

Some plants are balanced or neutral in themselves, but most plants bring us away from excess because of the balancing work they can do for the body. Generally, I use a plant that has characteristics opposite those of the illness I'm treating. Between the two (the illness and the herb), balance is found. For example, if the ailment is cold hands, use a plant that generates heat, such as ginger. If the cause of cold hands is poor circulation, look to an herb that promotes healthy circulation, such as strawberry, or to a nutritive herb such as viola to nourish overall health.

As the body moves toward balance, the herbal therapy needs of that body should be reevaluated. Perhaps the symptom of cold hands has disappeared. Is it because winter is over? Because circulation has improved? Each of us must heed our own body's signals and rhythms to determine the next step. Perhaps the use of ginger can be discontinued. Perhaps the dose of nutritive herbs can be reduced to a maintenance level, or discontinued for a time to evaluate the results.

Working Inside and Out

A common procedure in herbal therapy is to treat the ailment internally and externally at the same time. To relieve severe colic or gas pain, then, I might rest with a warm poultice of catnip tea on my stomach, as well as drinking frequent small sips of catnip tea.

No matter what any herbal expert may tell you, you know your body best. Herbal healing is an art. There is no one best way — only the way that works best for the individual. Ultimately, you must find your own balance, or it really is not balance at all.

There has been an increasing amount of research done lately on the old remedies used by people all over the world before the advent of Western medicine, but that work has far to go. Keep up to date in the research, and pay attention to any developments that might affect your home medicine making. Likewise, speak to your doctor before self-medicating with these herbal blends. There have been cases of people not taking their herbal medicine seriously enough to discuss it with their doctor — or being too shy to — and health problems getting worse instead of better, because the pharmacy medicines and the herbal medicines were in conflict with one another. That's no way to keep balance, now, is it?

Herbal medicine can be a powerful ally as you see your way through minor problems, like sore throats, loss of mental acuity, and tension. It can also work along-side conventional medicine, when carefully thought through. Horehound lozenges complement a prescribed medicated syrup for bronchitis, for instance, by soothing the immediate pain while the syrup works on the underlying cause. And if your gut is saying you should see a doctor about an illness, go to a doctor. Herbs may be potent, but so are bacteria, viruses, and mutating cells.

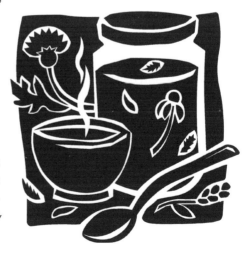

The Traditional Apothecary

Traditionally, the herbs in the following list have been used to treat ailments in a variety of ways. Check these in more detailed herbal sources to be sure there are no contraindications that apply to you and your state of health before embarking on an extended consumption routine.

- **Alfalfa leaves:** Treat digestive weakness, chronic inflammations, lost vitality.
- **Blackberry:** Used to treat dysentery and lesser causes of diarrhea. Roots are strongest, leaves and fruits milder.
- **Borage:** Restores strength to the recuperating, calms irritated tissues, reduces fever. Seed oil extract helps adrenal function and eases menopause and rheumatism.
- **Burdock:** Treats skin eruptions when applied externally (vinegar is best) and taken internally. A diuretic, it induces sweating and enhances liver function, helping to detoxify the body.
- **Catnip:** Calms nerves, soothes digestion, lowers fever.
- **Dandelion root and flower:** Diuretics that stimulate liver, reduce cholesterol, aid diabetes, stimulate digestion.
- **Garlic:** Reduces cholesterol, lowers blood pressure, regulates blood sugar, calms spasms, scares off parasites, and serves as an antibiotic and antiviral. Most of these applications require the garlic be raw, except for the cholesterol lowering.

Do Your Homework

Always research plants before you decide to make anything edible from them. Just because a plant is familiar, or even one you eat in some contexts, doesn't mean that it is safe for all uses. Nutmeg, for example, is commonly found in most kitchens, but it is toxic in relatively small doses. Every herbal cook should have ready access to a good, thorough herbal medicinal reference book.

- **Ginger:** Stimulates the circulatory system, thus energizing and bringing mental clarity and sharpness. Also soothes upset stomach and nausea and aids in recovery from colds and flu.
- **Horehound:** An old standby for sore throats, in syrups and lozenges.
- **Lavender:** Soothes tension, relieves headaches, stimulates appetite, uplifts.
- **Lemon balm:** Cooling herb, lowers fevers, alleviates bruises, cuts, and aches, speeds healing of sores, calms nervous stomachs.
- **Marsh mallow root:** Soothes mucous membranes, treating digestive disturbances and raw throats from coughs and colds.
- **Oat straw:** Soothes intestines, lowers cholesterol, fights nervous tension and anxiety.
- **Peppermint:** Cooling, stimulating, refreshing, induces light sweat, antiseptic (good for mouth rinses, wound washes, and sore throats), stimulates digestion, relieves nausea. And of course, pastilles for fresh breath!
- **Plantain:** Leaf used to treat external skin problems and internal digestive ones. Root used topically to heal stubborn skin wounds.
- **Poplar bark, buds:** Do not use if you can't take aspirin, unless the problem is stomach upset resulting from tablet use only, and don't give to children with a cold or flu. The active ingredient is much like that of aspirin, breaking up congestion. It's also used to treat rheumatism, headache, and weakness.
- **Raspberry leaf:** Used in teas to ease menstrual cramps and during pregnancy to prepare for delivery. Relieves diarrhea and skin irritations, too.
- **Red clover:** Sweet and cooling; rebuilds strength following flare-ups of allergies and arthritis, as well as during chemotherapy. With prolonged consumption, reduces blood's ability to clot — used positively to slow down arteriosclerosis, but should be avoided during pregnancy, around surgery, or if you have clotting trou-

bles. Take a day or two off its use each week for your body to recenter itself.

- **Rose:** Use only the small, busy, old-fashioned kind. Astringent and cooling, strongest when harvested as newly bloomed flowers.
- **Rose hips:** Full of vitamins C and E, traditionally used as a blood purifier.
- **Strawberry leaf:** Enhances circulation and well-being of the heart and blood vessels.
- **Thyme:** Boosts immune system; antiviral, antimicrobial, and antifungal. Apply tea in order to clean wounds, and drink it to calm stomach upset, cramps, and nervous problems. Avoid during pregnancy, as it may induce menses.
- **Violet petals, leaves:** Must be used fresh. Syrup preserves the flavor, makes a soothing throat relief. High in vitamins.
- **White pine needles:** Make into a drink or lozenges to loosen up congestion; most effective hot.

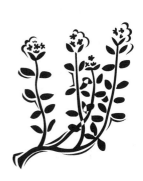

One Man's Meat Is Another Man's Poison

When trying a new plant, there is always the possibility of an individual allergic reaction. Simple and mild herbs are generally safe to test at home. First, rub a bit of the plant on a patch of skin. If no swelling or itching occurs in 24 hours, try drinking a small amount of tea made from that herb. Wait 24 hours before taking a larger dose. Some people find themselves allergic to many members of a whole family of plants. For example, people who are allergic to strawberry may have a similar reaction to rose hips or raspberry — all are members of the Rose family of plants.

Homespun Alchemy:
Making Medicinal Wine

Winemaking has been around far longer than those specialty home brewing supply shops that sell all kinds of paraphernalia, from fermentation locks to expensive and delicate yeasts, cadmium tablets, and even glass bottles and corks! Being a tightwad at heart, I wondered just how folks used to make wine without all that fancy equipment. Could I replicate the process in my own home?

I headed over to my local library to research an old English and Celtic form of wine called mead. What I found out was that not only were wines once made from a greater variety of fruits, but herbs were added as well to give unique flavors, scents, and healing properties. I have been hooked on winemaking ever since.

Making wine relies on the slow process of fermentation for preservation. Fermentation happens naturally as plants are left exposed to air and rot. While they do so, airborne yeasts and bacteria break down sugar and starch. Alcohol is excreted in the process. The yeast and bacteria keep producing alcohol, until eventually the environment becomes toxic to them and they die. This is what forms the sediment in your bottles of homemade wine and vinegar. The trick is to control this process to yield a desirable product.

It usually takes about 2 months to make a batch of wine from start to finish, but I actually put in only about 2 to 3 hours' effort in all. Fermentation can be smelled by every wild animal living in your county — they also consider wine a delicacy — so find a critter-safe area for your fermenting brew.

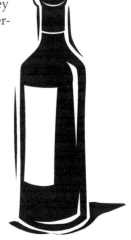

When starting out, you will probably want to produce several small experimental batches. Once you have your recipe down, you'll find it more economical to make larger batches. With experience, you're also likely to want to give the finished wine more time to age and mellow. Following are the proportions for both large and small batches. Note that the proportions are slightly different for the larger batch.

BASIC WINE RECIPE

For small, experimental batches:

1–2	quarts (1–2 liters) fruit (optional)
1½	gallons (6 liters) water
1	pound (450 g) honey (or other sugar source)
1	tablespoon (15 ml) baker's yeast
½–1	pound (200–400 g) herbs
1	pound (450 g) dried fruit

YIELD: ABOUT 1 GALLON (4 L) WITHOUT SEDIMENT

For larger batches:

4	quarts (4 liters) fruit (optional)
5	gallons (19 liters) water
3	pounds (1 kg) honey (or other sugar source)
1	tablespoon (15 ml) baker's yeast
3–5	pounds (1–2.25 kg) herbs
3	pounds (1 kg) dried fruit

YIELD: ABOUT 4 GALLONS (16 L) WITHOUT SEDIMENT

Equipment List for Making Wine

- Long-handled stirring spoon
- Paring knife
- Masher or grinder, to prepare fruit and herbs (optional)
- Large Crock-Pot or other container made of glass or stainless steel; or an oak barrel (I've even used a 5-gallon plastic bucket — not my first choice, but better than not making wine at all)
- Three or four 750 ml bottles for each gallon of wine
- Containers for siphoning
- Cheesecloth
- Rubber bands
- Plastic tubing

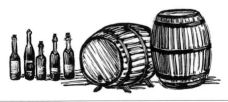

Step 1

Sterilize all the equipment you will use, including the containers for siphoning, with peroxide (see the box on page 4) or by boiling for 10 minutes.

Step 2

Gather your fruits and herbs of choice. Clean them, sorting out and disposing of any debris and moldy or diseased-looking pieces. Mash or cut the fresh (not the dried) fruit into 1-inch (2.5 cm) chunks. Cut any herb roots into 1-inch pieces or grind them coarsely. A food processor works well for this.

Step 3

Place all the fruits and herbs into a large ceramic crock or other nonreactive container. (Although many herbalists like to decoct and strain the herbs first, I find that even hard roots such as burdock yield their virtues through fermentation. I simply strain and press out the herbs at the end.) Add the water, honey, and yeast, but make sure your container is only three-fourths full to allow room for expansion. Stir until everything is fully combined.

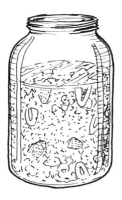

Step 3

Step 4

Cover with three layers of cheesecloth to allow the gases to exchange while preventing flies and renegade yeasts from getting in. Secure cheesecloth with a rubber band or string.

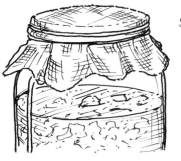

Step 4

Step 5

Set in a warm place (75° to 90°F, or 24°–32°C). Soon you will see bubbles start to rise. This is the start of fermentation, and means everything is working fine. After 5 to 7 days, you'll notice the fermentation process noticeably slowing down (the bubbling is less active but not altogether gone).

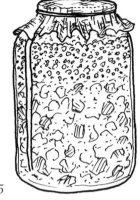

Step 5

Step 6

Add the dried fruit. Cover with clean cheesecloth. Let sit undisturbed until all fermentation (bubbling) stops — about 3 to 6 weeks, depending on the temperature.

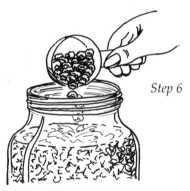

Step 6

Step 7

Strain all plant material out of the wine, using a press, a rice strainer, or a food mill to extract as much liquid from the plant material as possible. If you do not have any of this equipment, strain the wine through clean cheesecloth, then wrap the herbs in the cheesecloth and wring out the additional liquid. In larger batches, you may get as much as an additional gallon from this squeezing. Let the wine sit undisturbed in the original container or another large nonreactive container covered with clean cheesecloth for 24 hours to settle.

Step 7

Step 8

You will notice a layer of sediment on the bottom. Either decant the clear liquid slowly and then use a turkey baster to get the last bit out or set up a simple siphon.

To make a siphon you need two equal-sized containers and about 3 feet (90 cm) of ½-inch (13 mm) plastic tubing. Place the container holding the wine on a table and place the empty container on the floor. Fill the tube completely with water, pinching both ends to seal it. Hold one end over a sink or extra container at a lower level. Place the other end in the container holding the wine, then release the tube, allowing the water to flow out until the tube is filled with wine. Then pinch the end of the tube. Transfer that end into the empty container on the floor, and allow gravity to do its work. Monitor the siphon in the wine to make sure it does not get down into the sediment and start siphoning off that as well.

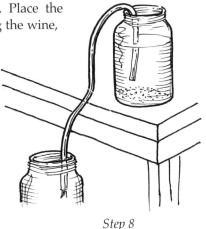

Step 8

Step 9

Pour the wine into sterilized wine bottles. I used to cork the bottles right away, but not anymore. If the fermentation isn't fully complete, the gas can pop the cork right out, leaving a big mess to clean up. To ensure complete fermentation, use a small deflated balloon as a test. Simply slip the balloon over the top of the bottle and watch for 24 hours. If there is any fermentation, escaping gas will inflate the balloon. Let the gas out of the balloon and keep testing until the balloon remains deflated for 24 hours. Then cork, label, and date the bottles. You can cover the cork with melted beeswax to ensure a proper seal and make it look more decorative.

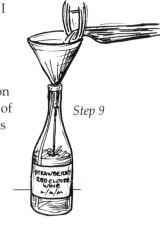

Step 9

Step 10

Store your wine in a cool, dark place for at least 6 months. This allows for harsh flavors to blend and mellow. Keep corked bottles stored on their sides; otherwise, the corks will dry out and there will no longer be a proper seal.

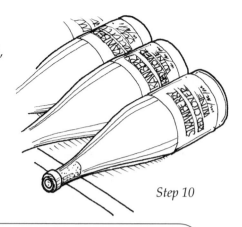

Step 10

Standard Dosage for Medicinal Wine

The standard dose for medicinal wines is 1 to 2 ounces (30–60 ml) taken one to three times a day, as needed. For children, I'll pour just-under-boiling water over the wine and let it rest for 5 minutes before serving. A little sweetener may be necessary.

My Favorite Medicinal Wine Recipes

Winemaking fosters the creative impulse — have fun mulling over all the possible fruit and herb combinations before making a batch. If you can't decide whether to make lavender-strawberry wine or lavender–rose hip wine, a good way to sample potential flavor combinations is to first make a small pot of tea from the ingredients and do a taste test.

I like to choose a fruit that has medicinal virtues suitable to the purpose of the wine. For example, for a wine designed to promote cardiac circulation, I would use the circulation-enhancing fruit strawberry instead of raspberry or blackberry. Just plug the following ingredients into the basic recipe on page 15.

WINE TONIC FOR IMPROVED CIRCULATION

Strawberry enhances circulation and thus the well-being of the heart and blood vessels. This formula will help to purify and revitalize the blood and circulation system.

For fruit:

Fresh ripe strawberries

For herbs, combine:

2 parts red clover blossom (nourishing herb with mild blood-thinning properties)
1 part alfalfa leaf (provides trace minerals)
1 part lavender flower (eases depression and aids digestion)
½ part violet blossom (gentle circulatory stimulant)
½ part whole crushed rose hips (rich source of vitamin E)

REJUVENATING WINE TONIC

This formula is especially good for rebuilding strength from exhaustion after pregnancy, from nursing, or after a long illness.

For fruit:

Raspberry, with 1 orange added per gallon (4 l) of water

For herbs, combine:

1 part violet blossom and leaf (nourishing, diuretic, and anti-inflammatory)
2 parts borage leaf (maintains adrenal health)
1 part lemon balm leaf (uplifts spirits)
1 part green oat straw, with developing seed heads (nourishes nervous system, soothing)
1 part alfalfa leaf (rejuvenating and nourishing)

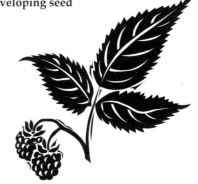

GARLIC WINE

Make just enough of this wine for 1 day's use, since it should be used fresh; many of the active principles in the garlic will be lost by the next day.

- **1 fresh garlic clove, crushed**
- **3 ounces (90 ml) wine**

Add the crushed garlic to the wine and let it rest for 10 to 15 minutes.

For external use: Apply this wine as a wash, or moisten a cloth with the garlic and lay on as a dressing.

For internal use: Sip the 3-ounce glass of wine slowly throughout the day.

The Origins of Garlic Wine

The use of garlic wine dates back to the Greek physician Dioscorides, who administered it to the Roman army. Dioscorides was also a famous herbalist, responsible for devising the method of cataloging medicinal items still used by modern pharmacists.

His list of recommended applications for garlic wine is impressive: treating chronic coughs, healing wounds cleanly, preventing infections, dispelling toxic poisoning from bites of bees and scorpions, preventing and eliminating internal parasites, preventing food poisoning, clearing the arteries, preventing the spread of infectious diseases, and as a disinfectant wash. Garlic poultices were used to treat wartime injuries all the way up through World War I, when they were applied as wound dressings, saving the limbs and lives of tens of thousands of soldiers.

Digestive Bitters

Bitters help balance overly sweet and salty diets. They activate digestive enzymes and bring warmth to the digestive process, helping the body break down and properly absorb the nutrients in our food. Most often they are used moderately in cooking or drunk just before eating.

BITTERS 1

For fruit:
> Apples, or an equal amount of apples and oranges, quartered

For herbs, combine:
- 1   part fall-gathered dandelion root (promotes secretion of bile and helps with digestive absorption)
- 1   part mallow root (soothing)
- 1   part burdock root (aids liver function)
- ½   part thyme leaf (stimulates digestion)
- ½   part lavender blossom (stimulates digestion)
- ½   part gingerroot — if you like a ginger "bite" and want a bitters that is aggressively warming (perhaps to balance a vegan diet), double the amount

BITTERS 2: DANDELION WINE

Dandelion wine makes an excellent digestive bitters all on its own. Take a 1-ounce (30 ml) serving of the wine 15 to 20 minutes before eating. It can also be taken after a heavy meal to aid digestion.

For fruit:
> 1 lemon and 1 orange per 1 gallon (4 liters) of water

For herbs:
> Dandelion flowers, picked early in the day

BITTERS 3

For children or those with sensitive, spasmodic stomachs.

For fruit:
>   Apples

For herbs, combine:
>   1   part catnip flower (calms nervous stomachs)
>   1   part dandelion flower (aids digestive process)
>   1   part mallow root (soothes irritated tissues)
>   1   part plantain leaf (soothes and heals)

Flower Wines

Basically any edible flower can be made into a wine. Some flowers are slightly insipid; adding a lemon will give their wines a little lift. You can also add a few walnut leaves for a drier, higher-tannin wine. One popular flower wine is, of course, rose petal, but lavender flower is equally sublime. A favorite of mine is blue wine made from borage, violet, and lavender flowers, with a couple of handfuls of crushed almonds thrown in for flavor. The wine will have the medicinal attributes of the flowers you choose.

Caution

Red clover leaf and blossom, along with other herbs that contain coumarin glycosides — these include strawberry, blackberry, and raspberry leaves — may form a toxic di-coumarol molecule when improperly dried. Di-coumarol reduces the blood's ability to clot. Pharmaceutical medicine uses it as a powerful anticoagulant. To avoid a potentially serious situation, always be sure to use only fresh or thoroughly dried and properly stored herbs for your wine- or vinegar-making process.

The leaves and seeds of apples, apricots, plums, cherries, and peaches contain a natural form of cyanide, hydrocyanic acid, which is released as that plant part is broken down. Do not add these leaves or seeds to your wine.

Medicinal Vinegars

On the day my daughter was due to be born, I thought I'd get ahead and make a big batch of strawberry wine before things got crazy with a new baby. I gathered strawberries that morning, and by lunchtime I had a 10-gallon crock filled and fermenting. Just when I thought I could sit back and relax, labor started.

Later that day an 8-pound baby girl was born! She was perfect in every way, and as babies will, she kept us hopping. But the wine turned out to be far from perfect. In my haste to make it, I hadn't sorted out the blemished strawberries, since they had all just been freshly gathered. Then I let the wine sit for several weeks before I finally got around to looking at it. When I took off the cheesecloth, the rapidly fermenting brew had turned to vinegar. My first thought was to throw it all away; it certainly wasn't useful as wine. But curiosity got the best of me and I let the brew finish fermenting. I strained it and decanted off the sediment — and ended up with a 5-year supply of the best strawberry vinegar this side of the Mississippi. It turns out that wine *wants* to sour. This is part of the ritual fermentation process. If you add fruit that is not sound, chances are good that bacteria are already present on it. I like making vinegar because I can use up otherwise discarded bruised peaches, apple peelings, and herb stems, thus extending the yield from my harvest.

Since producing my first unplanned batch of vinegar, I've found a few techniques to help ensure a good medicinal vinegar. On pages 26–27, you'll find a simple-to-make recipe that will ensure a good batch of vinegar.

Guidelines for Using Vinegars

Medicinal vinegars can be used in the same ways that the comparable herb wine would be used. They are excellent for people who are intolerant to alcohol. A tablespoon of honey and a tablespoon of herb vinegar in a cup of water makes a refreshing beverage — hot or cold — to help normalize digestion, restore the acid-alkali balance, and provide energy. Vinegars can be freely used internally and externally. And yes, you can use them on your salads — and how many medicines can you say that of?

Herbal vinegars are generally not as medicinally potent as their alcohol counterparts, but when made with herbs that nourish the organs such as alfalfa, violet, and red clover, herbal vinegars make a tonic superior to their counterparts. Tonics are a cornerstone on which to slowly build and maintain a healthy condition. They counteract nutrient deficiency, rebuild vitality, and should be mild and nourishing. Tonics are best taken daily and regularly. Herbal vinegars make a tasty addition to a diet, and their mild nature allows them to be used as a tonic. In fact, I keep taste foremost in mind when putting together a vinegar brew. Lavender, borage, violet, and rose all make sublime vinegars; the more culinary herbs such as ginger and thyme are great also.

It is difficult to determine the percentage of acid contained in homemade vinegars. Commercial vinegar is always 5 to 7 percent, and is strong enough to use as a preservative for pickling. Never use homemade vinegar to pickle vegetables or fresh herbs. The water content of the fresh plants may be just enough to tip the scale too far away from the acid content necessary to preserve the vinegar and prevent botulism from growing. Should you be concerned about a low level of acid, try adding a touch or two of 80-proof alcohol to enhance the preservation.

Although I have often read that medicinal vinegars don't last much longer than 6 months to a year in storage, I've not found this to be true of well-made home-brewed vinegars. A friend of mine recently used a 10-year-old bottle of home-brewed blackberry vinegar against an intestinal flu that had upset her whole family. She found it very viable indeed.

High-Calcium Brew

Vinegar is an excellent medium for carrying calcium into a formula. To make a high-calcium vinegar, incorporate herbs high in this nutrient such as alfalfa, fresh raspberry leaf, and red clover. Another good source is crushed and dried eggshells. Calcium will naturally leach into the vinegar solution until it reaches the saturation point.

BASIC VINEGAR

This recipe will make about 2 gallons (8 liters) of vinegar, without sediment.

2	gallons (8 liters) water
1–1½	pounds (400–600 g) herbs
2–3	quarts (2–3 liters) fruit
1	tablespoon (15 ml) baker's yeast
½	cup (125 ml) mother vinegar (see page 6)
1	pound (450 g) honey (or other sugar source)

1. Sterilize all the equipment you will use with peroxide (see the box on page 4) or by boiling for 10 minutes.

2. Gather your fruits and herbs of choice. Sort and discard any black or obviously molded parts of the fruit. A little bruising or discoloration (such as brown apple peelings) is fine, however.

3. Since the process of "souring" happens fairly quickly, take 1 gallon (4 l) of the water and use it to brew the herbs into a strong tea. Strain and press out excess tea from the plant material. Also, since the herbs are part of the vinegaring process, the resulting acid content is higher, decreasing the chance of spoilage. Add in the other gallon of water and let cool to room temperature.

4. In a 3-gallon (12 l) crock or other noncorrosive container, combine the 2 gallons (8 l) of room-temperature herb tea, fruit, yeast, mother vinegar, and honey.

5. Cover with three or four thicknesses of clean cheesecloth secured with a rubber band or string. Store in a warm place between 75° and 90°F (24°–32°C).

6. A key to making vinegar is exposure to air. Remove the cheesecloth and skim off any surface scum that may develop. Then give the brew a good stir (use a nonreactive, freshly sterilized spoon) once or twice a day for about a week. Skim off froth that rises from the stirring. Replace the cheesecloth cover when you're done stirring and skimming.

7. When the fermentation is finished, the bubbling will stop and the brew will no longer be frothy. It will smell and taste sour. This will take about a week. Strain out the fruit. Let settle overnight, covered with cheesecloth. Remove the cover and slowly pour off the clear liquid from the bottom sediment. Use a turkey baster to carefully get out the last bit of clear vinegar, or set up a simple siphon (see page

18). You can save the bottom sediment to act as the mother vinegar in your next batch of vinegar.

8. Pour the vinegar into bottles. Slip a small deflated balloon on top to monitor for possible fermentation. When the balloon remains deflated for 24 hours, fermentation has stopped. Now you may safely cork the bottles. Cover the cork with melted beeswax to ensure a proper seal. Label and date your bottles, and store them on their sides.

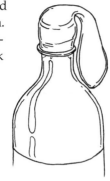

9. You can use the vinegar right away, but just like wine, the flavors of the herb vinegars mellow and blend with aging. Try to wait at least 3 months before using, if possible.

Step 8

Bittersweets: Making Syrups

In my opinion, jams and jellies cry out for a little herbal lift. Plain old strawberry rhubarb jelly is fine, but what if you added a touch of mint? or lavender? Yummm! What if you made a lavender syrup to use as a medicine — wouldn't that be yummy, too? Perhaps it is simply my sweet tooth speaking, but I get immense satisfaction from sharing with friends my homemade violet syrup on top of a big stack of cattail pollen pancakes. It is the best way I know of to turn another person on to the delights of herbalism. And I can make my family's medicine so tasty that it is easily disguised as food. Thus our food becomes our medicine.

Making Medicine Taste Pleasant

Syrups disguise the bitter or strong taste of herbs such as dandelion, white pine, raw garlic, and poplar bark. When a syrup is administered straight from the spoon, children don't notice the bitter until after they swallow the medicine. And somehow, the residual sweetness left in the mouth compensates for the bitter taste — enough so that my children, at least, always ask for another spoonful. Try medicinal syrups for anyone who simply cannot or will not tolerate a bitter or strong flavor.

Syrups excel at soothing sore throats, coughs, most digestive upsets, and sudden fatigue. However, their high sugar content makes them a poor choice for treating chronic fatigue, nutritive imbalances, and deep-seated chronic disorders such as diabetes.

A SIMPLE MEDICINAL SYRUP

I'll share with you a process that is by far the easiest way to turn any plain syrup into an epicurean feast. It's good for you, too.

    1   **cup (225 g) water**
    ½   **ounce (about 2 cups, or 550 ml) fresh herb leaves or flowers**
          OR
    ½   **ounce (about 2 cups, or 550 ml) herb roots or bark (reduce by half if using dry herbs)**
    1   **cup (235 ml) honey, maple syrup, rice syrup, or other sweet syrup**

1. Bring the water to a boil.

2. Remove from the heat and add the herb leaves or flowers. (If you are using root or bark, do not remove from heat, but allow to simmer over low heat until water is reduced by half.)

3. Let stand for about half an hour.

4. Strain out the herbs, reserving the liquid in a saucepan. You now have a very strong cup of tea.

5. Add honey or other syrup to the reserved liquid. Simmer over very low heat on the stove or in an electric warmer that maintains a temperature of between 90° and 100°F (32°–38°C) until most of the liquid is evaporated and the liquid is close in consistency to what the syrup was originally.

6. Bottle, label, and store in a cool, dark place or the refrigerator.

Faster Than Coffee

Try starting your day with a cup of instant zing. To make this concoction, add 1 tablespoon of homemade ginger-maple syrup to a cup (235 ml) of hot water. Add a squeeze of lemon. This delicious blend will help kick-start your day without leaving any caffeine jitters to follow.

AN EVEN SIMPLER SYRUP!

Here's an even simpler way to make syrup, using fruit jelly as the sweet base for your herbs.

1. Make ½ cup (120 ml) of a strong herb tea.

2. Mix tea well with 1 cup (235 ml) of fruit jelly of your choice. Apple jelly allows the flavor of the herbs to come through the most. Allow it to stand overnight in your refrigerator before using.

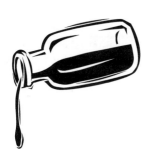

This is a good method to use if you are testing a new herb combination and uncertain about the flavor. I often try out any experiments this way before using them in a more complicated recipe.

Herb Jellies

You can also make a simple herb jelly by adding a cup of fresh, finely chopped herbs and flowers to a fruit jelly. Let stand overnight to give the flavors a chance to blend. It's a great way to incorporate fresh herbs into your diet — and even children will eat it!

Making Sugar-Free Syrups

Low-methoxyl-type pectin powders are derived from citrus peels and pulp. They can be used to make jams, jellies, and syrups that rely on calcium to bind and gel rather than sugar (like regular pectin jellies). You can usually find this type of pectin in health food stores: Pomona and Universal are two brand names to look for. When you open the box you'll find two packets, one with pectin, one with calcium. The calcium must be dissolved in water; a small amount of this mix is then added to the recipe.

Selecting Suitable Herbs

To make a syrup using a low-methoxyl-type pectin, it's best to use fresh and uncooked herbs. Fresh herbs help give a creamy texture to the recipe, while dried herbs merely seem gritty in comparison. Since the syrup is basically uncooked, delicate flower and herb essences are preserved — plus heat-sensitive vitamins like A and C will not be destroyed. For long-term keeping, however, you will have to store the finished product in the freezer.

Try this recipe with all manner of herbs and flowers: peppermint, rose, red clover blossom, lavender, lemon balm, violet — any pleasant-tasting herb or flower. You can even use hard fruits such as rose hips if you cut off the blossom ends of the hips first, then whir the hips in the blender with water until you get a milkshake consistency. Let stand for about 2 hours, then strain out the seeds through a sieve. Use this strained liquid to make your syrup. And of course there are all kinds of delicious fruits you can add to give an extra dimension to the flavor of the herbs. Try a lavender and orange-juice concentrate blend or apple-mint jelly to stimulate digestion. Rose petal, lemon balm, and strawberry is a centering, calming blend. Sweet cherry and lemon thyme syrup is sure to soothe a sore throat and ease coughs. Keep in mind how you will use the syrup as you create your recipes.

Working with Flowers

Flower petals like rose and dandelion are bitter at the base. When you gather them, pull up the petals in one hand and clip off the base with a pair of scissors held in the other. Preparing enough for a batch of syrup takes about 15 minutes — the same time allotted for a normal coffee break — and is infinitely more relaxing.

Use a pair of sharp scissors to clip the flower buds.

BASIC SUGAR-FREE SYRUP

2 cups (550 ml) fresh herbs, petals, or an herb-fruit combination
Lemon juice
1 cup (235 ml) water
1 teaspoon (5 ml) low-methoxyl-type pectin powder

1. Combine the fresh herbs, petals, or herb-fruit combination in a blender. Add lemon juice, ½ teaspoon (3 ml) at a time, to taste. Blend well. It may be necessary to add a little water to get the desired consistency, which should be like a milk shake. Remove from the blender and set aside.

2. Bring the water to a boil. Put it in the blender and add the pectin powder. Blend 1 to 2 minutes, until all powder is dissolved.

3. Add the blended herb mixture to the hot pectin mixture in the blender and process on low for 1 minute.

4. You do not need any sugar, but if you want to add sweetener for your own personal taste, do so now and blend on low until just mixed.

5. Add ½ teaspoon (3 ml) calcium water (from the envelope in the pectin mix). Blend again just enough to mix well.

6. Fill three 1-cup (235 ml) freezer-safe containers about two-thirds full and let them stand at room temperature for 1 to 2 hours. Store in the refrigerator, where the syrup will keep for about 3 weeks. If, when you go to use it, you discover that it has jelled too much, reheat it and add more water and herb (tea). If it hasn't jelled enough, reheat and add a little more pectin.

To save the syrup longer, you can freeze it; simply remove it from the freezer and let thaw for about an hour before serving.

To make jam: By adding a little extra pectin to this recipe, you'll end up with a wonderful no-cook freezer jam.

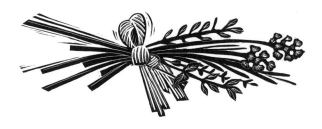

Other Storey Titles You Will Enjoy

Herb Mixtures & Spicy Blends, by Maggie Oster.
More than 100 flavorful recipes gathered from herb shops and farms across North America.
160 pages. Paper. ISBN 978-0-88266-918-2.

The Herbal Home Remedy Book, by Joyce A. Wardwell.
A wealth of herbal healing wisdom, with advice on how to collect and store herbs, make remedies, and stock a home herbal medicine chest.
176 pages. Paper. ISBN 978-1-58017-016-1.

The Herbal Home Spa: Naturally Refreshing Wraps, Rubs, Lotions, Masks, Oils, and Scrubs,
by Greta Breedlove.
A collection of easy-to-create personal care products that rival potions found at exclusive spas and specialty shops.
208 pages. Paper. ISBN 978-1-58017-005-5.

Herbal Remedy Gardens, by Dorie Byers.
More than 35 illustrated plans for easy-to-maintain container and backyard herbal gardens.
224 pages. Paper. ISBN 978-1-58017-095-6.

Herbal Vinegar, by Maggie Oster.
Dozens of recipes for vinegars that put herbs, spices, vegetables, and flowers to flavorful use.
176 pages. Paper. ISBN 978-0-88266-843-7.

Rosemary Gladstar's Medicinal Herbs: A Beginner's Guide.
How to grow, harvest, prepare, and use 33 of the most common and versatile healing plants.
224 pages. Paper. ISBN 978-1-61212-005-8.

These and other books from Storey Publishing are available wherever quality books are sold or by calling 1-800-441-5700.
Visit us at *www.storey.com* or sign up for our newsletter at *www.storey.com/signup.*